I Chose You
To Be My Mommy

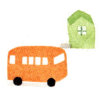

Director of Ikegawa Clinic
Author: Akira Ikegawa M.D., Ph.D.

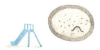

Futami Shobo Publishing Co.,Ltd

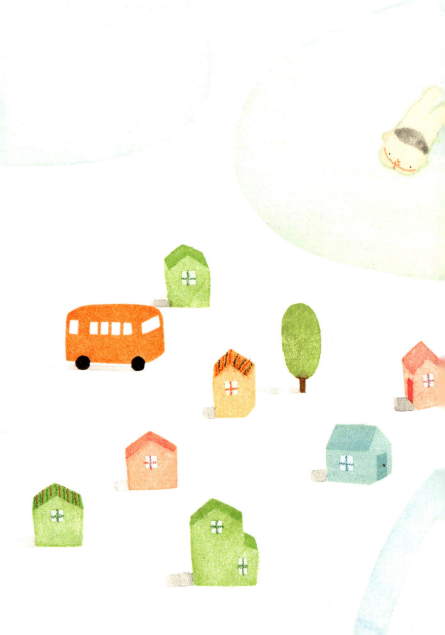

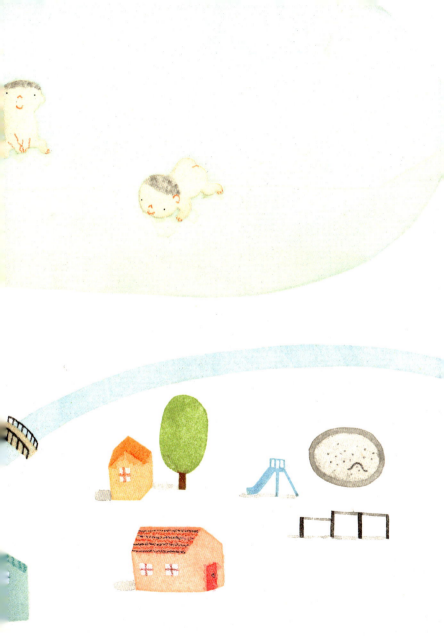

Foreword

....

Being in the mother's womb.

~ Remembering being born.

—Four years have passed since I started to study children's prebirth and birth memories.

It all started when I thought that if I were able to specifically find out whether "Babies are already conscious when they are in the womb", it might be useful for communication from pregnancy onwards. I surveyed 79 people, and the results were published in my previous book, "I Remember When I Was In Mummy's Tummy".

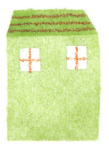
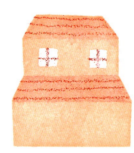
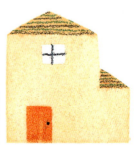

Ever since this book was published, many stories about prebirth memories and birth memories, not only from children but even from adults, saying

"My child told me this"

"In fact, I also remember something like this"

began pouring in to me.

Later on, I conducted a survey of more than 3500 people in total, with the help of daycare centers in Suwa City and Shiojiri City in Nagano Prefecture.

The results showed that more than 30% of the children who answered the survey had pre-birth memories, and approximately 20% of them had memories of their births.

(Details are provided at the end of the book.)

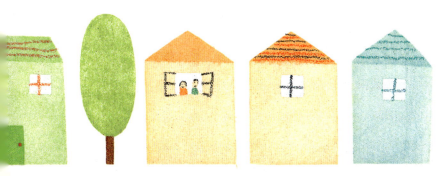

At first, they described their memories using expressions such as

"It was warm in the tummy"

"It was dark"

This was consistent with the findings published in my previous book.

But in the process of collecting many reports, I discovered that some children's memories went back even further, to before they entered their mother's tummy.

In full swing, some children began to relate their experiences, such as: What sort of place they were in before entering the tummy, how they came to choose their mothers and fathers, and as for the children who have brothers or sisters, some even talked about their future siblings…

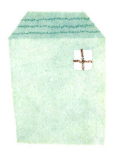
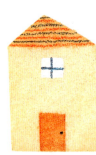
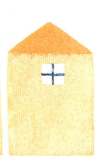
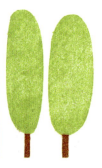

Though the children's ways of expression varied, they all had certain images in common, which were that the place they were in was warm, faintly light, a comfortable space; that there were some children just like them, and there were a few (or one) adults also; and when the time came, they chose their own mothers and fathers, by themselves or for a particular reason.

In this book, I mainly wrote about these,

"The memories before entering Mommy's tummy".

In the last half, I also wrote about the memories which bring out the feel of the bond of siblings and memories which some adults have managed to retain.

It's not a matter of whether to believe or not, I will be very glad if I can deliver the message that

"Children are thinking things such as these".

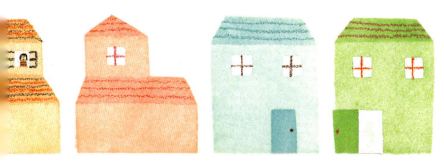

Illustration:
Kazue Takahashi

Translation:
Seika Smith

Book design:
Nobuko Oinuma

I Chose You

To be My Mommy

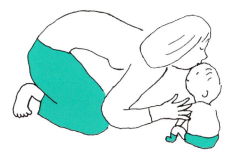

The ages given are the ages at the time when the children spoke of their memories.

It was dark inside Mommy's tummy, but it was warm,
and I was swimming.
I couldn't wait to see Mommy.
When I was born it was too bright.
When it's time to be born,
Somebody will let you know,
"Now you can go"
I couldn't wait for Mommy to hold me (in her arms),
But I was in a glass box.

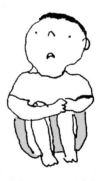

There were many kids in that country over there,

And we were watching from up above, saying

'that mommy looks pretty and kind' and things like that.

I made friends with some other boys, there were 3 of us,

We all thought it'd be nice to go to Mommy's place,

and I came to you, Mommy.

I picked you, because you are kind.

Yuhya Itoh / about 2 years old

From the time he started to talk until he was about 4 years old, he used to tell me this all the time. I was surprised because he couldn't have known that he had been in an infant incubator for several hours after his birth.

He always talked about "3 boys" even before our younger son was born, and I really ended up having 3 sons.

You know what? I was a light.

I had many friends of lights.

Great-Grandpa and Great-Grandma came to me,

and said, "the Nakahara family house is that one,

over there".

So I came.

Asahi Nakahara / about 4 years and 10 months old

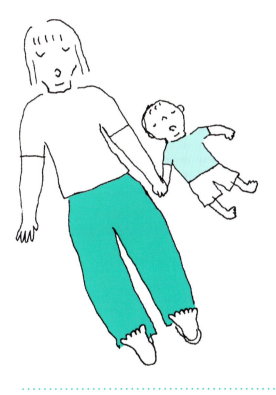

When we were taking a bath, I asked her, "What was it like inside Mommy's tummy?" This was her spontaneous reply.

I was with Sora (her younger brother) above the sky.

We were playing with a ball.

I told him, "I'm going first" and came.

I chose you, Mommy, because I wanted to be an actress.

Many stairs from the sky

were connected to many mothers,

but you were the prettiest, Mommy.

So I thought you could make me an actress.

When I came in,

you were holding out your hand to a mushroom

in a place like this, wearing clothes like this.

When I entered your tummy, Mommy,

there was a long cord,

I put it on my tummy.

It was easy.

Rina Tamura / about 5 years old

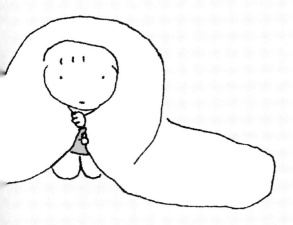

Before I ever heard this story, she asked me to let her join a talent agency.
The lessons were hard and I would have liked her to quit had she not told me this story. Until I heard this, I had felt like this child was "mine", but I learned that she came to me of her own free will, and since then my behavior towards her has changed to respect her as an individual.

You know what? I've been in the magic world before.

The magic world is bright, warm and comfortable.

When the sky tries to become night,

a wizard makes it morning.

There was something like a big pool.

The water there was warm,

and I swam really well.

There was a store called "The Whole Wide World"

Babies come there,

And from there they go away again with the wizard.

There are many babies in the magic world.

There are a few grown-ups, too.

The grown-ups don't have to work.

They're just watching over the babies.

(How did you come to Mommy and Daddy's home

from the magic world?)

The wizard brought me here.

We walked on a shiny warm road.

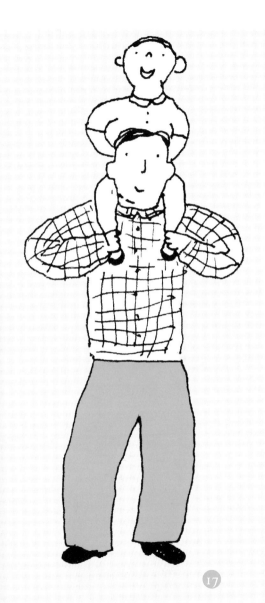

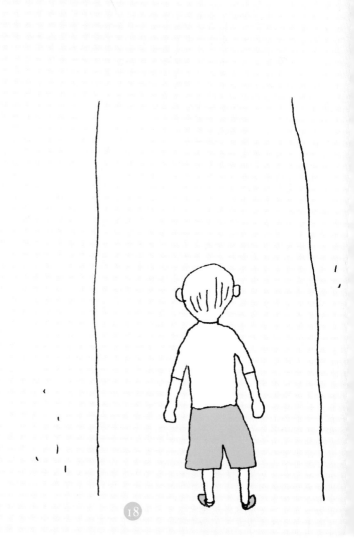

The road never branches off. It's straight,

and when you keep on going,

then you reach Mommy and Daddy's home.

At that time, there was a girl walking on the next street,

and I said to her "See you later!"

When I got sleepy, the wizard picked me up and flew.

Different babies go down different streets.

My street was just for me.

(Do you want to go to the magic world again?)

Yup!

But you know what?

I can't go to the magic world any more.

I can't go there at my age.

Tsubasa Kikuchi / about 4 years old

My son was looking at a Disney picture book; suddenly the picture of a wizard triggered him to splutter. I was surprised because normally he only talks of what exists in reality. Even today he sometimes talks about the magic world.

I picked Mommy and Daddy.
I was floating in the air with a grown-up guy
I didn't know,
Then we heard laughing voices from your house,
and the grown-up guy asked me if this house would do,
So I said yes.

Yasuo Yamada / 3 years old

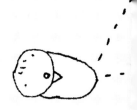

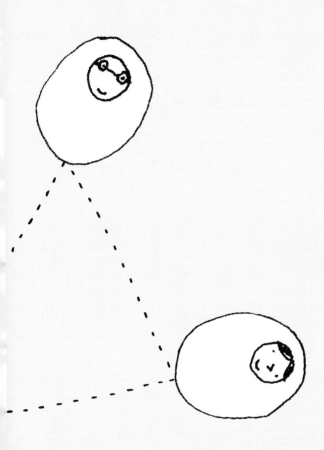

These are the words of my second son, who was 3 years old at that time, now he is 20. I was overwhelmed with marvelous and happy feelings and thanked him for choosing me and my husband.

(Where were you before you came into Mommy's tummy, Kuon?)
I was on the clouds.
There was a grassy plain over there.
(Were there any adults?)
No, no adults.
There are people who are like adults but they are all little.
We were tearing off pieces of clouds
and eating it together.

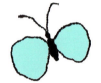

(Did you pick Mommy and Daddy, Kuon?)
Uh-uh, I didn't.
There was a grown-up guy at a place like a shop,
and he picked for me.

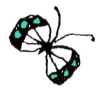

(Was Keito (his younger brother) there, too?)

Uh-huh.

I came whooshing in to your tummy first, Mommy,
then Keito came in next.

Then another baby came in.

(Was it a boy or a girl?)

A very active girl.

She was supposed to go to a different mommy,
but she didn't want to, so she followed me.

During yours and Daddy's wedding,
I could see you were holding hands.

I heard many people clapping their hands.

(You could see outside from the tummy?)

Uh-huh. I could see from the belly.

I saw ants and things.

(I wonder if the baby in Mommy's tummy can see right now, too?)
She can.
(Can you see the baby in the tummy, Kuon?)
I can't.
It's a special power that only the baby in the tummy has.
Don't you know that, Momma?
Once you come out, you lose it.

Kuon Morimoto / 5 years old

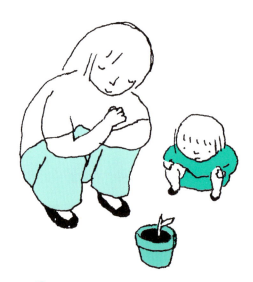

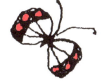

This was a conversation during breakfast. I was really intrigued, because he kept talking on and on although I had never discussed anything with him about heaven. I was surprised to find out that the baby I was pregnant with at that time really did turn out to be a girl. I believed he really could see from my stomach, because my husband and I had got married when I was pregnant with Kuon.

Above the sky, there is a bunch of kids this size,
and grown-ups about this big are taking care of us,
and little kids are looking down from the sky,
and we pick a house and we slide down there.
And so I decided to go where you were, Mommy.

At that time, I couldn't see Natchan (his younger sister),
but I think perhaps Natchan
decided to come to this house, too,
because Mommy and Daddy and I were here.

Atsushi Maki / about 3 years old

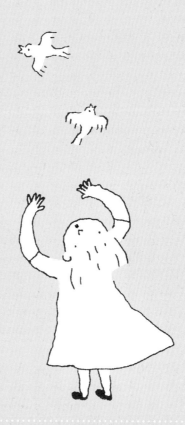

My son, now 9 years old, used to tell me this between the ages of 3 and 6 years. He told me about what it was like inside my tummy and before entering my tummy in great detail. But after starting elementary school, he began to say, "I don't remember that. Did I really tell you such a thing?"

(Mah-chan, what kind of place were you at
before you came to Mommy?)
Well, there were lots of kids there.
(Who else was there?)
A teacher.

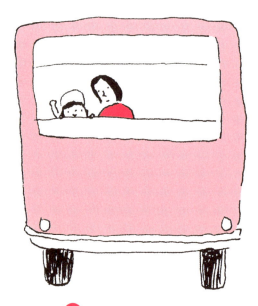

(What was the teacher like?)

Like the teacher from my daycare.

Ms. Sakai (the Principal) was there.

(Why did you come to Mommy and Daddy?)

Because I wanted to.

(Thank you for coming to us)

You're welcome!

Masanao Sato / about 3 years old

There was a period of time when my husband and I didn't get along, and I spent some uneasy days. This may explain why he was telling me about inside my tummy being "dark", "uncomfortable" and he told me "that's why I came out early." In fact, he was born by cesarean at 32 weeks.

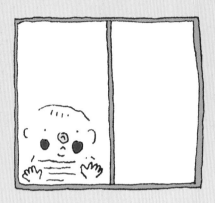

You know what? I was on a cloud,
and I was thinking,
ah, that house looks very nice,
they have big brothers, how nice, I wanna go there.
So I came here.
I'm glad I came.

Yoshiyasu Tsuchiya / about 2 1/2 years old

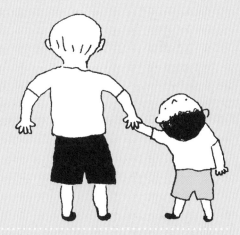

These are the words of my second son, who was then 2 and a half years old. He is now 23. He started to talk when he was 8 months old and he was always a chatty child.

Back then, I didn't quite understand what he meant, but several years ago

I learned about prebirth memories and thought "This must be what he was talking about."

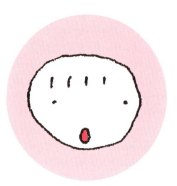

Know what?

The three of us decided we'd take turns coming here.

Sakura Gohongi / about 3 years old

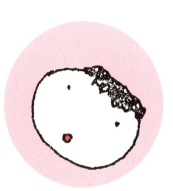

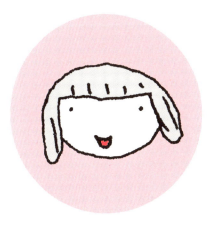

I'm the mother of 6 children, aged 11, 10, 8, 5, 3 and 1 years old. My eldest daughter told me this when I had my third child. I later wondered what happened to the three younger children. But thinking back, the third and fourth children are about 4 years apart and at the time, I was debating whether I should give birth to the baby, but now, I am truly happy that I did.

Yesterday, I went up to the sky,
and I saw a smiling baby there,
so I put it into Mommy's tummy.
Don't worry, Mommy.
The baby in your tummy is fine,
And it can't go back to the sky
without me,
So don't worry.

Yuhta Endo / 3 years old

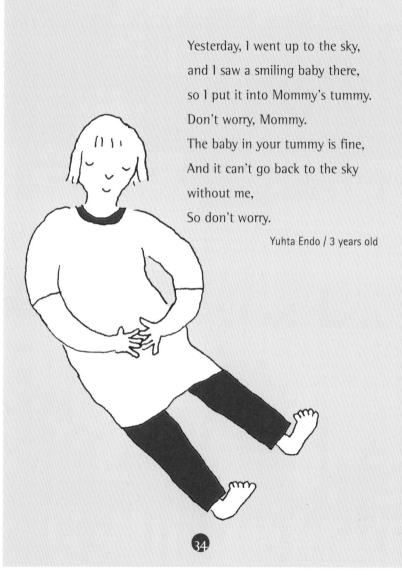

I was hoping for a second child, and I had been telling Yuhta, "I want you to go to the sky and bring back a baby for Mommy's tummy." It seemed that sometimes he would try at night; for about 3 months he kept telling me,

"there were only crying babies there, so there aren't any in your tummy".

And these were the words he told me one morning. I found out I was really pregnant that same month, and I thanked him many times.

But, when I was 2 months pregnant, I kept bleeding and my doctor told me that "the baby might not make it". Then Yuhta spoke those second words to me, when I was filled with anxiety. Soon after that, my unborn baby appeared to me in a dream and told me, "Don't worry. I will be born alright. A smiling big brother has been to see me."

Why is the baby leaving?

(Well, the baby came into Mommy's tummy,

but it's gone now, back to the clouds.)

(Staring at my stomach) It's still in there.

(Eh? Is it?)

It's still in there but it's saying it will be leaving soon.

(Will you ask it to come again?)

Uh-huh, I will.

(...will you, please?)

I already did.

(Did it say anything?)

It said thank you.

(Really? Will it come again?)

Uh-huh, it said it will.

(I wonder when...?)

Well, when it gets warm and the tulips bloom...

She will come again.

The baby's a girl.

Gakuto Mochizuki / about 2 years and 10 months

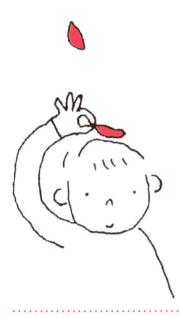

I had had a miscarriage, in which the fetal heart beat had stopped at 2mm.
This was the conversation I had with my son when we came home after crying for an hour. I was surprised but at the same time I felt calm, as if all the tension had drained away from my shoulders.

(Do you remember being in Mommy's tummy?)

...Uh-huh.

(What was it like?)

...Like a refrigerator

(Was it cold?)

Uh-Uh, it was warm.

(Did you stay still in Mommy's tummy?)

...I was playing with a big brother and big sister.

(Yeah?

Was the brother about Rui (her 6-year old cousin)'s age?)

Uh-uh, he was even older than that.

The big sister was about Rui's age.

(Let's send the big brother in the refrigerator

back to the clouds.)

No!

I wanna go up in the clouds, too.

(Don't go, because Mommy will miss you.)

OK, I won't.

(To my stomach) Big brother,

Go back to the clouds.

You don't have to worry, OK?

Yurika Torigoe / 3 years old

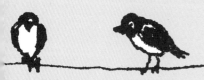

These were the words of my daughter, whom I had 15 years after I married.
To tell the truth, I had been pregnant twice before: in the year I got married and another 10 years after that, but I had miscarried both babies in the second month. I wonder if she was playing in my stomach with her two siblings, who were never born.

Before I was born, I was something like an invisible ball
so tiny you couldn't see me,
and I was playing around jumping, in a place
like a universe with no stars.
I wasn't happy or sad.

From there, before I knew it, I became like a long worm,
there were hundreds of us, bumping shoulders and stuff.
It was crazy!
But in the end, I was the only one left.

And one day all of a sudden, my body started to grow.
Everyday, I grew and grew soooo fast. .

At first, I was like a killifish; I looked just like a baby pig,
my eyelids were very thick.
After a while, my eyelids got thinner,
and then I could see the light from outside.
When my fingers were done, I would play,
rubbing my fingers and toes and doing somersaults.

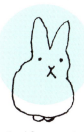

Inside your tummy it was purplish red and
it was kind of slimy but firm, like a pot,
I could hear a sound like running water
and a throbbing sound.
Inside was soft and cushiony,
and there was lots of warm water in there.
I curled myself up.
There was a long string coming from my belly button
that joined me to your tummy.

When my body got really big, suddenly,

your tummy started to move and pushed me out.

When the exit got this big,

I went into a mysterious tunnel.

The mysterious tunnel would move by itself

and push me out.

Inside the tunnel was stringy,

And my shoulders were caught in it

and it took quite a while. It was a bit tight and hard.

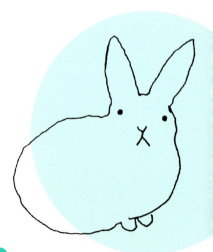

At first it pushed me, but

it was hard because I had to get out by myself in the end.

I didn't have a problem breathing.

When I got closer to the exit,

the skin got thin and I could see outside through it.

When my head started to come out,

I could open my eyes better,

And when I came outside, my eyes opened right up.

I didn't want to cry but my body started to cry by itself,

and then, I closed my eyes.

Issui Yamamoto / 7 years old.

He had been saying things like this since he was 3 years old, and when he was 6 years old, he even drew pictures about it. He talked in the most detail just after he turned 7. Now at the age of 9, he seems to remember only about 30% of it.

I remember being in a place like a cloud before I was born.

The place was lit by a light,

It felt like I was riding on a ball of mixed colors of pink,

green and white.

It was fluffy and comfortable.

As I was with female friends,

I was asked, "Who would you like?"

by someone who was like a great King,

so I chose my mother.

My friends chose mothers who were far away.

When I was coming down into my mother's tummy,

I was with some of my friends,

but one of them said "I'm tired so I'm going home"

and went back.

She said that she would go to the same mother again.

Yukiko Arai / 20 years old

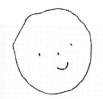
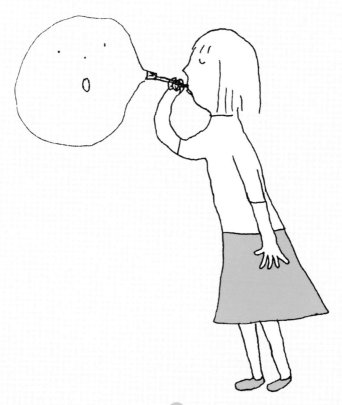

I have my own prebirth memory.

I've had this ever since I was a small child.

To put it briefly, the place was comfortable. It was dark.

When I was sleeping comfortably,

I heard a voice out of nowhere saying,

"It's nearly time to go. Wake up."

But I was so sleepy, and said, "Wait a little bit more."

and I fell asleep again.

My next memory is that though I was sleeping,

I was pulled from my back,

and pushed out to somewhere bright and cold.

When I was in the upper grades of elementary school,

I found out I was born by cesarean section.

I heard it was 2 weeks past the due date.

I remember things from birth till I was one year old,
and I also remember things before I was born.

There were fields and fields as far as the eye could see.
It was neither hot nor cold; I didn't get hungry,
time passed slowly,
and it was a very tranquil place. But I was also quite bored.
There was a tunnel like a well,
and from there you could go to the human world.
When you die, you go back there again.
Though you can get into the well freely,
it is thought that we are sent to the human world
for a kind of "life training'.
We experience hardships as well as joys, you know.
Our prebirth memories are supposed to be erased
while we're going down the tunnel.
But I wished, "Please don't let me forget".
For some reason, I've remembered wishing such a thing.

Noriko Masubuchi / 40 years old

Postscript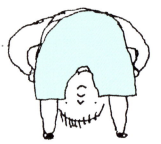

My previous book "I Remember When I Was In Mommy's Tummy" was written based on a survey which was conducted in the year 2000 about prebirth memories.

The survey showed surprisingly that 53% of the children answered that they did have prebirth memories, and 41% of the children answered that they remembered being born. I was amazed at the high numerical value.

However, this survey's population was small: just 79 people. In fact, I handed the questionnaire to many more people, but this was the number of responses that I received.

I wondered if 53% was an accurate figure; I wonder how

things are in a practical sense—. In order to find out, I began to want to conduct the survey on a scale of about a thousand people. Although I had a hard time finding facilities where I could ask for cooperation on such a large scale, in August 2002, 1773 parents of children from 18 daycare centers and kindergartens in Suwa City, Nagano Prefecture and two other daycare centers/ kindergartens agreed to cooperate.

At the time of the 2000 survey, "prebirth memories" were known only to some people, and most people's reactions were of complete puzzlement. But this has changed so much in the last several years. The idea of "prebirth" has become quite normal among the general public.

Of 1773 parents, 838 (47%) responded to the survey. Of these, 34% (288 children) had prebirth memories, and 24% (197 children) remembered being born.

Furthermore, in order to confirm these figures, I also asked 1828 parents of children from 19 daycare centers in Shiojiri City,

Nagano Prefecture in December, 2003. The response rate was 43%, with replies received from 782 parents.

This time, 31% (243 children) reported having prebirth memories, while 18% (137 children) remembered being born.

Though this was less than half, it became clear that around 30% of the children did have prebirth memories.

Having come this far, I was finally able to confirm my suspicions that babies already know many things when they are in the womb, and they remember them even after they are born.

In the Shiojiri City survey, I had asked some more detailed questions. First, of the children who answered that they had prebirth memories, only 20 children had "talked about it on their own", while an overwhelming number of 223 children had "talked about it when asked".

Come to think of it, I recently heard a story like this.

I heard that at a certain kindergarten, they read the story "I

Remember When..." to the children, and when it was over, the children started talking about their prebirth memories saying, "I also...", "Me, too...", as if they were discussing completely normal events.

I think it is possible that they just hadn't talked about it previously because there had been no need to, or no one had asked them before, and many more children might consider their prebirth memories to be the most natural and normal thing in the world.

The period of time when they speak of these memories also shows a trend.

This starts when they are a little over one year old, when they start talking, and reaches a peak when they're between 2 and 4 years old. After 5 years of age, the memories seem to fade rapidly.

In fact, many people have said things like "when he was 2 or 3 years old, he told me about it many times but now at the age of 4, he doesn't even remember ever talking about it."

But, there are some children who still remember after this period of time. In this survey, I also asked parents about their own memories, and 16 out of 1407 people (1%) who replied to the survey said that they still retain these memories. When I asked the same question at a lecture, about one in 100 people raised their hands, so I realized that adults also have these memories at around that rate.

I am trying to figure out what can be ascertained from these "prebirth memories", "birth memories" and "memories before entering the womb," what we can perceive from this, and what I can do as an obstetrician and gynecologist.

Although there are still many things to be clarified, I think probably the following three things can be surmised from these results:

(1) Parents are chosen by their children.

(2) Children are born to lend support to their parents.

(3) Children are born to accomplish their own goals.

The words of the children in this book illustrate the first point. While most of the children represented in this book "chose their mommy and daddy by themselves," there were also cases in which the children chose to have someone else make this decision for them."

As for the second point, this is what I feel and realize as a parent every day myself, and there are children who clearly state this.

I heard that little Kuon, who appears in this book (page 22) had said when he was 5 years old, "when I was in Mommy's tummy, she was coughing a lot and I thought it wasn't good. So I was cleaning hard in Mommy's tummy."

He said "cleaning" meant getting rid of his mother's gloomy feelings, her tiredness and getting bad food out of her body to make it clean.

I have heard children say several times that they were "cleaning in the tummy", "the baby's cleaning right now", looking at the baby in the tummy from outside. I now see what they meant.

Also, there are children who clearly say "I was born to make mommy smile", "I came to help mommy".

Regarding the third point, although there have not been many children who have verbalized their goals, this is the impression I've been getting.

We can see an example in the words of little Rina who "came (here) to become an actress" (page 14) and Ms. Masubuchi (page 46) who says "although the world before birth is pleasant, it doesn't satisfy the spirit of challenge and adventure. I came to this world to experience many things."

Children are born with their own goals. Parents have their own purpose in life also. I think parents should support their children so that they will accomplish the goals they have at birth, and at the same time, they should live positive lives.

Investigation by Questionnaire Regarding Fetal/Infant Memory in the Womb and/or at Birth

Akira Ikegawa, Administrative Director of Ikegawa Clinic

ABSTRACT

The purpose of this study is to clarify the possession rate of fetal/infant memory in the womb and/or at birth and to validate its characteristic. A total of 1620 answered questionnaires of the 3601 distributed were returned, giving an overall recovery rate of 45.0%. The possession rates of womb and birth memory were 33.0% and 20.7%, respectively. Parents, too, responded with regard to their own memory from birth, and 1.1% appeared possessing such memory. The possession rate is relevant to the mother's feeling and speaking to the fetus during pregnancy, and irrelevant to the irregularity in delivery. Most memories were positive.

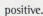

KEY WORDS: memory, womb, birth, fetus, infant, oxytocin, cortisol

INTRODUCTION

From the 1980's there has been awareness of the existence of fetal/infant memory in the womb and/or at birth through research by a number of researchers such as Thomas R. Verny, M.D., David B. Chamberlain, Ph.D., etc. They conducted the research using the hypnotherapy method. However, detailed study on the ratio of existing fetal/infant memory in full consciousness has not been conducted yet. The objective of this research is to investigate fetal/infant memory in full consciousness. When pregnant mothers came to my clinic with their child/children for antenatal care, I asked them whether their child/children carried some memory related to their birth. This has been asked regularly since 1999. It turned out that many children possessed such memory, though some mothers hesitantly described their children's talk. At that time, the mother seemed to think that her child's memory was just funny talk and at this point, I thought that it was imperative to investigate the fetal/infant memory closely. How many children really possess such memory? As the possession ratio of fetal/infant memory had not been investigated yet, I decided to set up an investigation, for the purpose of which, a clearly defined group of population would be examined.

In this investigation, memory in the womb has been defined as the memory of the embryo/fetus while still in the womb; memory at birth as the memory of the fetus/neonate before, at or after birth; and fetal/infant memory has been used with reference to both memory in the womb and/or at birth. As a result, I was able to distribute a questionnaire to be answered by mothers/fathers of 3,601 children at nursery schools in two different areas. The questionnaire focused on questions about fetal/infant memory possessed by children, and also included some questions about fetus/infant memory possessed by parents themselves with regard to their own birth.

METHODS

This investigation by questionnaire consisted of two parts and was conducted in Japan. The first part was carried out at 17 nursery schools in Suwa-City (population about 52,000), and two other local kindergartens during the period of August and September,

2002. The second part was carried out at 19 nursery schools in Shiojiri-City (population about 65,000) during the period of December, 2003. These two parts were combined and the results were used in this research.

Questionnaire Items

The questionnaire consisted of the following items:

- The mother's age
- The child's age
- Whether the child had talked about a memory in the womb and/or at birth.
- The age at which the child talked about a memory for the first time.
- Sex of the child
- If there was a memory, whether the child had talked about it after the mother's asking, or had volunteered.
- If there was no memory, whether the child simply had no recollection, or had refused to respond.
- Whether the mother tried to communicate with the fetus during pregnancy.

- If the mother tried to communicate, whether the child had a memory about it.
- Whether the mother had a stress-free, pleasant pregnancy.
- Whether, according to the mother, her delivery had been smooth or difficult.
- Whether the delivery was vaginal or with Caesarean section (with labor pain present or not).
- Whether the delivery had been carried out using vacuum extraction or forceps extension.
- Whether uterotomica had been used.
- Whether there had been breech presentation.
- Whether there had been coiling of the cord.
- Whether the parents had a memory from their own birth.

Statistical analysis based on chi-square test was used to assess the results.

RESULTS

Recovery Rate of the Questionnaire and Other Particulars

A questionnaire for the first investigation at Suwa-City was distributed to 1,773 parents, and the total of 838 answered questionnaires were returned, giving a recovery rate of 47.3%. The second questionnaire at Shiojiri-City was distributed to 1,828 parents, and 782 answered questionnaires were returned, giving a recovery rate of 42.8%. A total of 1620 questionnaires were answered of the 3601 questionnaires that were distributed, giving an overall recovery rate of 45.0%. The minimum number of children per nursery school was 16, and the maximum number was 210. The average number of children per nursery school was 93, in the total of 38 nursery schools. The mean average age of mothers who gave a response was 33.7 ± 4.4 (mean ± S.D.) years, and that of the children was 4.0 ±1.4 years. The age at which the majority of the children reported a fetal/infant memory, was between 2 and 3 years. Two of the children demonstrated some fetal/infant memory by means of gesture, after the parents questioning, at the age of 10 months (Fig.1). As for the gender of children possessing fetal/infant memory, there was no significant difference, with womb memory being reported by 268 boys and 254 girls, and birth memory by 174 boys and 156 girls.

Figure 1 - Child's age at which Fetal/Infant Memory was Recognized or Hinted at for the First Time

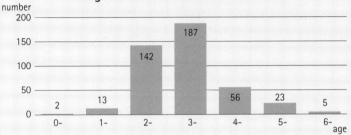

Possession Rate of Fetal/Infant Memory

The number of children who reported memory in the womb and at birth was 534 and 335 respectively, with corresponding memory possession ratios of 33.0% and 20.7%, of the total number of 1620 responses to the questionnaire (Table 1). 38 children of 534 who reported womb memory (7.1%), had volunteered to talk about the memory, while 496 children responded after questioning (92.9%), which is equivalent to 2.3% and 30.5% respectively, of the total number of questionnaires answered. 22 Children of 335 who reported birth memory (6.6%), had volunteered to talk about the memory, while 313 children responded after questioning (93.4%), which is equivalent to 1.4% and 19.3%, respectively, of the total number of questionnaires answered (Table 2).

Table 1 – Possession Rate of Womb Memory/Birth Memory

Memory	Present	Not present	Unclear	Total
In the womb	534 (33.0%) 45.1%*	649 (40.1%) 54.9%*	437 (27.0%)	1620 (100%)
At birth	335 (20.7%) 30.9%*	748 (46.2%) 69.1%*	537 (33.1%)	1620 (100%)

Note.* The number indicates the ratio when excluding the "unclear" cases.

Fetal/Infant Memory in Adults (Possession Rate)

The possession rate of memory in adults was examined through questions addressed to the parents (Table 3). 16(1.1%) parents of 1,407 (774 mothers, 633 fathers) who responded with regard to their own memory, reported fetal/infant memory. Among mothers, there was no one who reported simultaneously existing memory in the womb and at birth. Among fathers, two persons reported having both memories simultaneously.

Possession of Fetal/Infant Memory was Unconfirmed

There were three types of responses in the group where fetal/infant memory could not be confirmed. These were the "refused to answer", "child was not asked", and "child's response unclear". The details and conditions of "refuse to answer" were unclear. The number of cases where the child "refused to answer" was over 50%

of the unconfirmed cases for both memory in the womb and at birth (Table 4). The ratios of "refused to answer" cases for memory in the womb and/or at birth based on the total number of responses (1620) were 15.4% and 16.8%, respectively. Many of the cases where the "child was not asked", were due to the child's not being able to talk yet.

Table 2 – Details of the Children Possessing Fetal/Infant Memory

Memory	Volunteered Responses/1620	Responses after questioning/1620	Combined responses/1620
In the womb	38 (7.1%) 2.3%	496 (92.9%) 30.5%	534 (100%) 33.0%
At birth	22 (6.6%) 1.4%	313 (93.4%) 19.3%	335 (100%) 20.7%

Table 3 – Parents Possessing Fetal/Infant Memory

Memory	Present	Not present	Total
Mother			
In the womb	5 (0.6%)	769 (99.4%)	774 (100%)
At birth	5 (0.6%)	768 (99.4%)	768 (99.4%)
Father			
In the womb	3 (0.5%)	630 (99.5%)	633 (100%)
At birth	5 (0.8%)	625 (99.2%)	630 (100%)

Communicating with the Baby during Pregnancy

"Committed" in Table 5 refers to the group of mothers who tried to communicate with the fetus during pregnancy actively, and "indifferent" refers to the group of mothers who rarely or never tried to communicate with the fetus during pregnancy. When mothers tried to communicate with the fetus during pregnancy, there appeared a tendency of existing fetal/infant memory. Similarly, commitment during pregnancy significantly affected response in the way of an increase of the "refused to answer" cases.

Table 4 – Possession of Fetal/Infant Memory Unconfirmed

Memory	Refused to answer/1620	Child was not asked/1620	Child's response unclear/1620	Total/1620
In the womb	249 (57.0%) 15.4%	178 (40.1%) 11.0%	10 (2.3%) 0.6%	437 (100%) 27.0%
At birth	272 (50.6%) 16.8%	242 (45.1%) 14.9%	23 (4.3%) 1.4%	537 (100%) 33.1%

Table 5 – Effect of Parents' Attitude with regard to Communicating with the Fetus during Pregnancy on the Possession of Womb/Birth Memory

Communicating with the fetus	Memory in the womb			Memory at birth		
	Present	Not present	Refused to Answer	Present	Not present	Refused to Answer
Committed	290 (41.4%)	263 (37.6%)	147 (21.0%)	184 (27.5%)	317 (47.5%)	167 (25.0%)
Indifferent	207 (34.2%)	336 (55.4%)	63 (10.4%)	125 (21.9%)	382 (66.8%)	65 (11.4%)
	P<0.00001			P<0.00001		

Mother's Evaluation of a Smooth/Difficult Delivery

When a mother considered her delivery to have been a difficult one, memory in the womb tended not to be present (p=0.02589). However, birth memory did not appear to be influenced by the mother's assessment of her delivery (Table 6). When the mother assessed her delivery as smooth, the child's memory in the womb and/or at birth tended to be positive, and conversely, it tended to be negative, when the mother assessed her delivery as difficult, but there was no significant difference (Table 7).

Table 6 – Effect of Mother's Feeling with regard to Smooth/ Difficult Delivery

Delivery	Memory in the womb		Memory at birth	
	Present	Not present	Present	Not present
Smooth	340 (44.0%)	433 (56.0%)	221 (31.2%)	488 (68.8%)
Difficult	111 (52.6%)	100 (47.4%)	71 (36.8%)	122 (63.2%)
	P=0.02589		P=0.13925	

Table 7 – Assessment of Children's Memory with Respect to Smooth/Difficult Delivery

Delivery	Assessment of memory in the womb		Assessment of memory at birth	
	Positive	Negative	190 (96.4%)	Negative
Smooth	230 (95.8%)	10 (4.2%)	221 (31.2%)	7 (3.6%)
Difficult	72 (91.1%)	7 (8.9%)	59 (89.4%)	7 (10.6%)
	P=0.18603 using Yates' correction		P=0.05847 using Yates' correction	

Memory in cases with Irregularity in Delivery

The irregularity in delivery, such as, vacuum extraction, forceps extension, use of uterotomica, breech presentation, and/or coiling of the cord, did not appear to influence the possession of memory in comparison with normal vaginal delivery. The rate of the possession of memory in the cases of Caesarean section appeared to vary regardless of the existence of labor pain (Table 8). There was no actual correspondence between the mother's assessment of her delivery as difficult or smooth and the medically assessed irregularity of delivery.

DISCUSSION

If newborn babies are capable of retaining memory in the womb and/or at birth, we should reconsider our attitude with regard to childbearing management. Many studies have been done to submit evidence of fetal memory. However, it can be hardly said that obstetricians are convinced about the existence of fetal/infant memory still now. This study was not designed to prove the existence of fetal/infant memory. It is really difficult to prove fetal memory at this point, though, among others, Chamberlain has also made reference to the possession of birth memory among the young and adults in his articles (Chamberlain, D. 1988/1989). This study was designed to confirm the possession rate of fetal/infant memory based on child response. After search of related articles, I came to the conclusion that there must have been no survey previously conducted on the possession rate of fetal/infant memory.

Table 8 – Possession of memory in cases with Caesarean section

Labor pain	Memory in the womb		Memory at birth	
	Present	Not present	Present	Not present
Present	14 (51.9%)	13 (48.1%)	8 (27.6%)	21 (72.4%)
Not present	40 (58.0%)	29 (42.0%)	19 (30.2%)	44 (69.8%)
	P=0.586861		P=0.995726 using Yates' correction	

The Possession Rate of Fetal/Infant Memory

From the results of this study, the possession rate of womb memory was 33.0% and that of birth memory was 20.7% (Table 1). The results indicate that one-third of the children possessed memory in the womb and a quarter of the children possessed memory at birth. This research indicates the possession ratio in children up to 6 years old. The age at which the majority of the children who began to talk about fetal memory was between 2 and

3 years, and at the age of 6 years the number decreased significantly (Fig. 1). If research had been limited to the ages of 2 to 3 years, the possession ratio of memory might have been higher.

Why Don't We Notice the Fetal/Infant Memory?

If many children possess fetal/infant memory, why don't we notice? It can be considered to be due to two possible reasons. One of the reasons is that few children (only 1-2%, Table 1) are likely to volunteer to talk about their early memory, and another is the disbelief with which ordinary parents tend to treat the possibility of their child possessing such early memory, and as a result the unlikeliness of their trying to confirm such a memory with their child. The possession rate decreases with age and this is particularly shown in another unpublished research I have conducted at elementary schools and junior high schools in Japan, according to which the possession rate of fetal memory was around 5-9% and 1-4%, respectively. In this research, it was moreover proved that 1.1% of the adults also possess early memory from their own birth (Table 3). Considering all various factors together, the fetal/infant memory does not always disappear on reaching a certain age, but it might be held up to even adult age, though, as naturally expected, it gradually diminishes.

The Factors that Contribute in Retaining Fetal/Infant Memory

The following hormones are known as factors affecting memory: oxytocin, cortisol, serotonin, corticotrophin releasing factor (CRF), cholecystokinin, adrenocorticotropic hormone (ACTH), etc. Verny has shown that oxytocin is an important factor in extinguishing memory and also that the stress hormone cortisol is known to extinguish the recall of traumatic memories, thus playing a protective role during stress (Verny, T. 1981/2002). The stress hormone ACTH acts to carry on memories. Gulpinar and Yegen have reported that the peptides cholecystokinin, serotonin and CRF play strategic roles in the modulation of memory processes under stressful conditions (Gulpinar MA, Yegen BC, 2004).

Table 7 indicates fetal/infant memory, assessed as positive or negative. In most of the cases it is positive, regardless of the mother's assessment of her delivery as difficult or smooth, which suggests that unpleasant memories tend to be erased. However, when stress exceeds a certain level, secretion of the protective hormones may not be sufficient to provide protection, and as a result unpleasant memories may be retained. In the present research the trigger point of the stress level at which the protection system fails to resolve, has not been defined. Also the type of memory, positive or negative, was independent of the mother's assessment of a difficult or smooth delivery. It is difficult to justify why possession rates of memory in the womb and memory at birth, were different by about 10% because there may be many factors participating. One possible factor may be the length of the stimulation period. Memory in the womb may be relatively easy to be retained by repeated stimulation for periods as long as a pregnancy. On the other hand, memory at birth may be relatively hard to be retained because the duration of the event of childbirth is very short compared to a whole pregnancy period. The memory may be easier to be retained with repeated stimulation. Another possible influencing factor in the decreased possession rate in memory at birth, may be the protection mechanism which acts to extinguish agony experience at birth by secretion of oxytocin and other hormones. There is no significant difference in possession rates of memory in the womb and memory at birth between cases with labor pain present (increase levels of released oxytocin at birth) and cases without labor pains (reduced levels of released oxytocin at birth). Table 8 suggests that the lower levels of oxytocin is an influencing factor in the retaining of womb memory, as the memory possession ratio for cesarean section cases without labor pain is 58.0%, which is slightly higher than that of the cases with labor pain present.

The attitude of the parent who does not talk to the fetus during pregnancy, may be creating unpleasant conditions for the fetus, in which case the child tends to efface both memory in the womb and at birth (Table 5). The stressful condition experienced by the fetus during pregnancy may have a direct connection to the observed decrease in the rate of retained memory at birth due to secretion of oxytocin, cortisol and other hormones. In the laboratory it has been observed that oxytocin and cortisol efface memory. In table 6, why does the possession rate of memory in the womb tend to increase in the difficult delivery group? Heinrichs M. and co-worker indicate that central oxytocin selectively influences memory performance depending on the kind of memory test used and the psychobiological relevance of stimuli (Heinrichs M., Meinlschmidt G., Wippich W., Ehlert U., Hellhammer D.H., 2004). Oxytocin may act to reduce unpleasant feelings, while pleasant feelings are less influenced. Since with breast-feeding oxytocin secretion is sustained, the puerperal woman may forget the labor pains she has experienced.

How the "Refused to Answer" Group is Regarded

About 15% of the children in this study who refused to answer were considered to be likely to have retained fetal/infant memory. The pattern did not show a consistent tendency with the mother's general feeling with regard to her pregnancy. It will be necessary to further investigate the background and the details of this group in a future study of fetal/infant memory.

Is Fetal/Infant Memory Influenced by the Irregularity in Delivery?

It is generally believed that there is a tendency to retain fetal/infant memory in difficult deliveries. In this study, the irregularity in delivery, such as, the use of vacuum extraction, forceps extension, or uterotomica, breech presentation or coiling of the cord, did not influence the memory possession rate in comparison with the cases of normal vaginal delivery. There was hardly any difference in memory possession rates of memory at birth between easy and difficult delivery cases, but there was a significant difference for memory in the womb (Table 6). Memory in the womb was retained when mother assessed her delivery as difficult.

Does Antenatal Training have an Influence on the Retaining of Fetal/Infant Memory?

The importance of antenatal training has been known since the ancient times. Mother talks to the fetus naturally. However, recent mothers in Japan tend to ignore their fetus and/or they are not inclined to talk to their fetus. This study shows that memory in the womb and at birth is retained when the mother talks to the fetus. There tends to be a higher possession rate of memory in the womb in the difficult delivery cases compared with the smooth delivery cases, but the fetal/infant memory is usually positive in most children. This indicates that the possession rate of fetal/infant memory is certainly directly related to the mother's feeling during the pregnancy period and at delivery. Therefore, it is important to take notice of the mother's feeling and to maintain a good mood during pregnancy and at birth. There is a strong suggestion that antenatal training can influence fetal/infant memory, in which case it is important that pregnant women remain conscious of such fact and show their affection during pregnancy.

CONCLUSION

In this research, about 30% of the children less than 6 years old possessed fetal/infant memory, and about 1% of the adults had their own fetal/infant memory, which leads to the naturally expected observation that the possession rate of fetal/infant memory decreases with age. The possession rate is undoubtedly influenced by the mother's feeling and speaking to the fetus during pregnancy and moreover, positive memory tends to be retained in children, more than negative memory. With these points in mind, it becomes evident and suggestive that we should politely handle childbirth based on the premise of existence of memory in the womb and/or memory at birth.

REFERENCES

Chamberlain, D. (1988) Babies remember birth. New York: Ballantine Books.

Chamberlain, D. (1998) The Mind of Your Newborn Baby. Berkeley, CA: North Atlantic Books.

Gulpinar M.A., Yegen B.C. (2004, Dec): The physiology of learning and memory: role of peptides and stress. Curr Protein Pept Sci. 5 (6), 457-473.

Heinrichs M., Meinlschmidt G., Wippich W., Ehlert U., Hellhammer D.H. (2004, Oct). Selective amnesic effect of oxytocin on human memory. Physiol Behav. 30; 83 (1): 31-8.

Verny, T., and Weintraub, P. (2002). Pre-Parenting Nurturing your child from conception. New York: Simon&Schusdter.

Verny T., Kelly J., (1981) The Secret Life of the Unborn Child. New York: Dell Publishing.

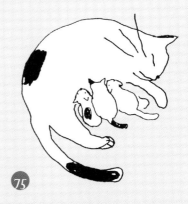

[About the Author] Akira Ikegawa

Dr.Akira Ikegawa was born in Tokyo Japan in 1954. He is a Doctor of Medicine. He graduated from Teikyo University Medical School.After working in obstetrics and gynecology at the Ageo Central General Hospital as the head director, he established the Ikegawa Clinic in Yokohama in 1989. In September 2000, he reported about "fetal memories" at the Joint Medical Seminar of the Japanese Medical and Dental Practitioners for Improvement of Medical Care, and this report was introduced in newspapers.Today, Dr.Ikegawa hopes to help people lead meaningful lives through childbirth.

*If you or your children have "fetal memory", please contact our clinic by Fax or e-mail.
Ikegawa Clinic2-5-13, Daidou, Kanazawa-ku, Yokohama City, Kanagawa Pref. 236-0035 Japan
Tel: +81-45-786-1122 / Fax: +81-45-786-1125 / e-mail: aikegawa@jcom.zaq.ne.jp
Prenatal Memory Network http://prenatalmemory.net/en/

I Chose You To Be My Mommy

2016年11月30日　初版発行

著者　　　池川　明 Akira Ikegawa

発行　　　株式会社二見書房
　　　　　東京都千代田区三崎町2-18-11
　　　　　電話 03(3515)2311［営業］
　　　　　　　　03(3515)2313［編集］
　　　　　振替 00170-4-2639

印刷　　　株式会社堀内印刷所

©Akira Ikegawa 2016, Printed in Japan ISBN978-4-576-16208-9
http://www.futami.co.jp
＊本書は2006年7月に出版された本の新版です。
This is a new edition of a book published in July 2006.